Patient Satisfaction and Dr. Burnout
The Long View
Your 22nd Psychiatric Consultation
William R. Yee M.D., J.D.
Copyright applied for March 14, 2021

Introduction

Recently I was advised that there were a series of patients reporting dissatisfaction with my treatment.

I was not given the patient's names or the basis for their dissatisfaction.

All I knew is that one patient had reported to a therapist that she was dissatisfied with my treatment because I would not prescribe Lunesta.

This could be any of my patients because I inform all my patients on the first visit that I do not prescribe addicting medications because like all facilities, all neighborhoods, there is an epidemic of alcoholism and drug addiction.

Lunesta is addicting and has the additional FDA warning against next day drowsiness. I rely on:

[5-15-2014] The U.S. Food and Drug Administration (FDA) is warning that the insomnia drug Lunesta (eszopiclone) can cause next-day impairment of driving and other activities that require alertness. As a result, we have decreased the recommended starting dose of Lunesta to 1 mg at bedtime. Health care professionals should follow the new dosing recommendations when starting patients on Lunesta. Patients should continue taking their prescribed dose of Lunesta and contact their health care professionals to ask about the most appropriate dose for them.

FDA Drug Safety Communication: FDA warns of next-day impairment with the sleep aid Lunesta (eszopiclone) and lowers recommended dose.

Because any medication can cause drowsiness the next day, on the first contact I give all my patients a written handout that states that if the patient is drowsy while driving a police officer can give them a ticket for impaired driving under the influence of the medication. I also give patients written advice that the officer may see small children in the car and be required to report to Child Protective Services to put the children into Foster Care.

Lunesta, and the other Z Drugs all have the following FDA warning:

FDA adds Boxed Warning for risk of serious injuries caused by sleepwalking with certain prescription insomnia medicines.

FDA Drug Safety Communication

"[04-30-2019] The Food and Drug Administration (FDA) is advising that rare but serious injuries have happened with certain common prescription insomnia medicines because of sleep behaviors, including sleepwalking, sleep driving, and engaging in other activities while not fully awake. These complex sleep behaviors have also resulted in deaths. These behaviors appear to be more common with eszopiclone (Lunesta), zaleplon (Sonata), and zolpidem (Ambien, Ambien CR, Edluar, Intermezzo, Zolpimist) than other prescription medicines used for sleep."

"As a result, we are requiring a Boxed Warning, our most prominent warning, to be added to the prescribing information and the patient Medication Guides for these medicines. We are also requiring a Contraindication, our strongest warning, to avoid use in patients who have previously experienced an episode of complex sleep behavior with eszopiclone, zaleplon, and zolpidem."

The Long View: My Fifty Years

My medical education started in 1968 at the age of twenty-one.

I attended Bible School at the age of four and learned the Golden Rule, treat others the way you would have them treat you.

I am Chinese and Swedish and multicultural by DNA and family environment.

My favorite class in college was a class in Social Anthropology that explored the many ways that different cultures manage child rearing, marriage, social relationships, law and other cultural issues.

After completing medical school, I swore the Hippocratic Oath to do no harm.

In training as a psychiatric resident, I was educated in psychoanalysis including the concepts of transference, countertransference and resistance to treatment.

I was trained in Freudian analysis, Jungian analysis, Rogerian analysis, Adlerian analysis, Horneyian analysis, etc.

I learned about the oral, anal, phallic, latent, and genital stages of psychosexual development of maturation from birth to adult life.

I learned about unconditional positive regard from the Rogerian school of psychoanalysis

I learned about birth order, social and cultural issues from Alfred Adler's school of psychoanalysis.

I learned about women's issues from Karen Horney's school of psychoanalysis.

I learned about social issues from Erich Fromm's school of psychoanalysis.

Medical ethics requires that:

1. I respect the patient
2. I listen to the patient
3. I am transparent with the patent
4. I educate the patient
5. I promote patient autonomy

What does medical ethics mean in practice?

Respect means that I make accommodations to the patient's culture, gender, and preferences.

I ask patients if they want a chaperone, the door open or closed, if they want counseling, medication, or both. How often they want to be seen, if they have suggestions for improving service, if they are satisfied with treatment, when they want to see me next. It is always the patient's choice.

Listening to the patient is more perception than reality.

To accommodate patients' perceptions, I ask them if they want me type their words into the note word for word as they speak, or if they want me to write a summary after the face-to-face meeting is completed.

Some patients have the perception that I am not listening to them even though I am typing their statements word for word into the progress note.

Other patients prefer that I type their statements word for word into the progress notes because they do not want any distortions of their statements to be part of the medical record.

You can have one, but not both, unless you tape record the interview. Unfortunately, I do not have the equipment to tape record my interviews with the patients.

I am transparent with the patient. I advise the patient as to my role.

6. I am an expert witness for the court.
7. I am an expert witness for the plaintiff.
8. I am an expert witness for the defendants.
9. I am the personal physician of the patient.
10. I have obligations to report child abuse to child protective services.

11. I have obligations to report crimes to various authorities.
12. I have obligations to report threats to various authorities.
13. I offer medications that reduce symptoms by 20% to 40% on average in one out of every three or four patients treated.
14. I advise the patient that more than fifty percent of patients stop taking medications or don't fill their prescriptions for medications.
15. I rarely cure mental illness and I cannot refer the patient to a psychiatrist who usually cures mental illness.
16. I recommend that meditation, aerobic exercise, sleep hygiene, meditation, deep breathing, relaxation, stimulus desensitization, EMDR, Cognitive behavior therapy and other alternatives before starting medications.
17. I recommend that the medications are started at a low dose to minimize side effects.
18. I recommend that the medications be titrated up slowly to allow for the body to adjust to the medication side effect.
19. I recommend that the medication be used only as a temporary treatment

until symptoms are adequately controlled by alternative treatments or remit.

20. I advise the patient that I will start the medications with or without alternative treatments after advising the patient to exhaust the alternatives first.

21. It remains the patient's decision whether or not to take medications.

22. It remains my duty to educate the patient as to the risks and benefits of alternative treatments.

23. I will offer one medication after another until the patient has had the opportunity to try them all or feels that medications are a waste of time.

Medication noncompliance is greater than fifty percent and is 75% according to some research.

I rely on

Pediatric Psychotropic Medication Compliance: A Literature Review and Research-Based Suggestions for Improving Treatment Compliance
Sabine Hack and Byron Chow
Journal of Child and Adolescent Psychopharmacology Vol. 11, No. 1Articles

Published Online: 5 Jul
2004https://doi.org/10.1089/1044546017501434
65

And

Psychotropic medication non-adherence and its associated factors among patients with major psychiatric disorders: a systematic review and meta-analysis
Agumasie Semahegn, Kwasi Torpey, Adom Manu,1 Nega Assefa, Gezahegn Tesfaye, and Augustine Ankomah
Syst Rev. 2020; 9: 17.
Published online 2020 Jan 16. doi:
10.1186/s13643-020-1274-3
PMCID: PMC6966860
PMID: 31948489

On the first face to face appointment, I give the patient a six-page printout about the treatments of mental illness.

This is because there is too much information to remember and not enough time according to current practices in brief therapy.

I promote patient autonomy.

At every point it is the patient's choice:

24. Do you want a chaperone?
25. Do you want the door opened or closed?
26. Do you want me to type every word you speak or write a summary after the face-to-face appointment is completed?
27. Do you want psychotherapy, medication, or both?
28. Do you want to see me weekly or on some other schedule?
29. Do you have suggestions on how I can improve my services?

I have been the medical director of two mental health centers.

I have done annual performance evaluations of residents in training, medical doctors, and psychiatrists under my supervision.

Evidence- based medicine is the Gold Standard of Medical Care.

In medicine, and particularly in psychiatry, evidenced based medicine is an imaginary construct because the research is of low quality and not reproducible

The dilemma of annual performance evaluations is that science does not provide tools for performance evaluation beyond attendance and completion of paperwork.

I rely on:

1,500 scientists lift the lid on reproducibility
Survey sheds light on the 'crisis' rocking research.
Monya Baker
NATURE | NEWS FEATURE
25 May 2016 Corrected: 28 July 2016

And

Bad papers are still published. But some other things might be getting better.
By Kelsey Piper Oct 14, 2020, 12:20pm EDT

As a medical director I was confronted with this dilemma.

If I gave a substandard performance evaluation, I was admitting that I could not hire competent psychiatrists and doctors.

If I gave a substandard performance evaluation, I was admitting that I could not train medical students, psychiatric residents, doctors, and psychiatrists that had been successful all their lives until they came under my supervision.

To make things worse the weakness in research did not offer me tools for training or performance evaluation that are evidenced based.

Let us explore the psychiatric research to examine the state of the art on March 13th, 2021.

This research has the goal of determining what the physician can do to improve patient satisfaction.

The converse is to identify physician behaviors that contribute to patient dissatisfaction.

There are many studies examining the basis for patient satisfaction.

These studies have been inconclusive and offer contradictory results that invalidate any claim that patient satisfaction is based upon specific factors.

The research on patient satisfaction does not support any sound basis for determining the cause of patient satisfaction and patient dissatisfaction.

The operant fact is that person-related characteristics have been found to be both determinants and confounders simultaneously and not reliable as a basis of determining the basis for patient satisfaction and dissatisfaction.

I rely on:

Determinants of patient satisfaction: a systematic review
Enkhjargal Batbaatar, Javkhlanbayar Dorjdagva, Ariunbat Luvsannyam, Matteo Mario Savino, Pietro Amenta
A Perspect Public Health 2017 Mar;137(2):89-101. doi: 10.1177/1757913916634136. Epub 2016 Jul 20.
PMID: 27004489 DOI: 10.1177/1757913916634136

Patient safety and clinical effectiveness are positively related to patient satisfaction which is not related to characteristics of the physician.

I rely on:

A systematic review of evidence on the links between patient experience and clinical safety and effectiveness
Cathal Doyle1, Laura Lennox1,2, Derek Bell1,2
Published by the BMJ Publishing Group Limited.
Volume 3, Issue 1

The operant thought in this article is that patient satisfaction is an imaginary construct without validity on a scientific basis. The basis of patient satisfaction remains to be identified by research and remains debatable.

I rely on:

A systematic review of patient and caregivers' satisfaction with telehealth videoconferencing as a mode of service delivery in managing patients' health
Joseph F. Orlando ,
Matthew Beard ,
Saravana Kumar
Published: August 30, 2019
https://doi.org/10.1371/journal.pone.0221848

My experience is that doctor burnout is a product of increasing the patient caseload, increasing the documentation requirements, and reducing the time available to complete the assigned tasks.

This is a universal experience in all employment situations to reduce costs and increase cash flow. This is a simple equation.

In the article below Burnout was defined by the following factors:

1. overall burnout
2. emotional exhaustion
3. depersonalization
4. personal accomplishment

Associated with physician burnout were:

1. depression and
2. emotional distress

The operant work products of physician burnout are:

1. unprofessional behaviors
2. unsafe care
3. low patient satisfaction

4. depersonalization

What is unprofessional behavior?

Professionalism and unprofessionalism are to sides of the same coin and subject to many definitions by many writers.

The article below adopts four abstract concepts which are also subject to various definitions and therefore remain artificial constructs. They are:

1. excellence
2. accountability
3. altruism
4. humanism

As these are abstract concepts professionalism was further defined by the following factors to approximate professionalism:

1. adherence to treatment guidelines
2. referrals to treatment or other services
3. malpractice claims
4. poor communication practices
5. low empathy

What is low patient satisfaction?

1. Patient reported satisfaction and
2. perceived enablement scores

What is depersonalization? The authors below relied on the Maslach Burnout Inventory™ (MBI) to define depersonalization:

1.lack of empathy

    a. Unfeeling engagement with the patient
    b. impersonal engagement with the patient

While being trained in psychoanalysis the psychiatrist is trained to be neutral in response to avoid shaping the patient's thoughts and feelings. It can be argued that by giving positive responses the psychiatrist is molded into a codependent in prolonging the illness. The positive responses by the psychiatrist can be experienced as a reward for being mentally ill, thereby prolonging the mental illness through positive reinforcement.

If a facility has a common problem with protracting and enhancing mental illness such as PTSD, then it is incumbent upon the facility to look at the corporate culture and what common factors enhance and prolong the PTSD.

I rely on:

Association Between Physician Burnout and Patient Safety, Professionalism, and Patient Satisfaction
A Systematic Review and Meta-analysis
Maria Panagioti, PhD; Keith Geraghty, PhD; Judith Johnson, PhD; et al, Anli Zhou, MD; Efharis Panagopoulou, PhD; Carolyn Chew-Graham, MD; David Peters, MD; Alexander Hodkinson, PhD; Ruth Riley, PhD; Aneez Esmail, MD, PhD
Original Investigation Physician Work Environment and Well-Being
September 4, 2018
JAMA Intern Med. 2018;178(10):1317-1331. doi:10.1001/jamainternmed.2018.3713

Although research on Team Based Care reveals some benefit. The suboptimal quality of research requires better research to confirm and clarify the actual benefits and costs.

I rely on:

Can Team-Based Care Improve Patient Satisfaction? A Systematic Review of Randomized Controlled Trials
July 2014PLoS ONE 9(7):e100603
DOI: 10.1371/journal.pone.0100603
Source Pub Med

Now let us examine patient dissatisfaction.

Patient dissatisfaction is associated (caused?) by the following:

1. ineptitude
2. disrespect
3. waits
4. ineffective communication
5. lack of environmental control
6. substandard amenities (6.9%).

I rely on

What can we learn from patient dissatisfaction? An analysis of dissatisfying events at an academic medical center
By: Alicia V. Lee, MD, John P. Moriarty, MD, Christopher Borgstrom, Leora I. Horwitz, MD, MHS
J. Hosp. Med. 2010 November;5(9):514-520 | 10.1002/jhm.861

Politics can be an issue among medical staffs in various organizations.

Political skills are as important as medical skills.

Is building your brand important? The following four attributes are important in a medical career:

1. likability
2. achievements
3. connections/friend at work
4. political skills.

I rely on:

Hospital Politics Don't Have to Be a Dirty Business
MICHAEL SILVERMAN, MD and DREW WHITE, MD, MBA ON OCTOBER 10, 2017
Copyright © 2019 EPMonthly.com

I suppose the takeaway is that the physician must

1. keep up with his medical education with Continuing Medical Education to maintain licensing and medical staff appointments.
2. Sustain political activities to maintain his brand among the medical staff.

Who determines which physician is "problematic" in the Medical Staff?

Is it the:

30. Hospital CEO?
31. Hospital Executive Committee?
32. Hospital Peer Review Committee?
33. Chief of the Medical Staff?
34. Departmental Chairmen?
35. Medical Staff Peer?
36. Anonymous Other?

Since politics are a part of every medical staff there are many issues that may start the process of reviewing a physician for "problematic," behavior.

There are many issues that make a Medical Staff Member, "problematic":

37. Criminal Behaviors.
38. Drug and Alcohol abuse.
39. Abuse of Staff and Patients.
40. Whistle blowing.
41. Patient complaints and low satisfaction ratings.
42. Cultural Differences in practice style.
43. Eccentric Documentation.
44. Eccentric Referral Patterns.

Hospitals, Medical Staffs, and Medical Staff Members have created problems for themselves by "corrective actions," addressing the, "problematic physician." The following are some of the problems based upon my personal experience and review of the literature:

45. Lawsuits with money judgments for wrongful termination.
46. Lawsuits with money judgments for defamation.
47. Lawsuits with money judgments for violation of 42 U.S. Code § 1983;
48. Lawsuits with money judgments for violation of 42 U.S. Code § 1985;

49. Hospital records seized by United States Marshals and made public records.
50. Prosecution for criminal activities.
51. Subjected to additional reviews by the Joint Commission.
52. Loss of Joint Commission Accreditation.
53. Bad press and loss of community confidence.
54. Congressional investigations and interventions.
55. Change of Facility Chain of Command from the CEO on down.
56. Loss of immunities for failure to comply with statutory time limits.

The Health Care Quality Improvement Act of 1986 -H.R.5540 — 99th Congress (1985-1986) was designed to provide guidelines for managing medical staff, protecting medical staff rights and offering immunities for the medical facility managing medical staff in "good faith."

Let us dissect the following:

"Provides protection from liability under Federal and State laws for members of a professional review body and their staffs who, in the reasonable belief that the action was in the furtherance of quality health care, warranted by the facts known, and after a reasonable effort to obtain the facts, take actions which adversely affect the clinical privileges or professional society membership of a physician. Provides such protection to those who provide information to professional review bodies."

The physician subject to an adverse action by the "professional review body and their staffs"

What is the professional review body?

The physician's attorney will argue that the "professional review body" includes, but is not limited to:

57. The Facility CEO
58. The Facility Executive Committee
59. The Facility Pharmacy Committee
60. The Facility Credentialing Committee
61. The Facility Peer Review Committee
62. The Facility Medical Records Committee
63. The Physician's supervisor
64. The chain of command between the Physician's supervisor and the CEO
65. Any other Facility employee or officer that intersects the physician and that physician's activity at the Facility.

Let us dissect the concept of reasonable belief.

What is a "Reasonable Belief?"

The physician's attorney will want to know what are the facts that form the "reasonable belief?"

66. Who alleged that the physician's conduct was defective?
67. What was the allegation?
68. What was the motivation for making the allegation?
69. Did the person who made the allegation have a history of other allegations?
70. Were there similar allegations by others?
71. When was the physician notified of the defective conduct?
72. What was the physician's response to the allegation?
73. Which individual or Committee investigated the allegation?
74. What are in the records of that investigation?

Let us dissect, "the reasonable belief," that are warranted by the facts known:

The attorney for the physician will want to know:

75. "What is the reasonable belief," that supports your action?
76. What are the facts that support your, "reasonable belief?"
77. What are alternative "reasonable beliefs," based upon these facts?
78. What were the physician's stated reasonable beliefs?
79. What was your basis for not accepting the physician's "reasonable belief"?

Let us examine "furtherance of quality health care,"

80. How does your "reasonable belief," serve the best interest of the facility, patients, and the affected physician?
81. What are viable alternative "reasonable beliefs"?
82. How do the alternative "reasonable beliefs" serve the best interest of the facility, patients, and the affected Physician?

Let us dissect "reasonable effort to obtain the facts":

83. What did you do to obtain the facts?
84. When did you make the effort to obtain the facts?
85. When did you contact the affected physician?
86. What did you tell the affected physician?
87. What was the affected physician's response?
88. What was your effort to confirm the affected physician's response?
89. In what ways were your efforts different from prior practice?
90. Is there a possibility that the allegations were mistaken?
91. Is there a possibility that the allegations were false?
92. Are you convinced that your investigation was thorough and without bias of any kind?

Let us dissect the actions taken that adversely affect the clinical privileges or professional society membership?

1. How were similar allegations against other physicians managed?

2. What corrective actions were offered to the physician?

3. When were the corrective actions offered to the physician?

4. What were the alternative actions available to the individual or committee?

5. Why was the action taken rather than the alternative actions?

6. What was the practice with prior physicians in regard to corrective actions?

7. Are you sure you eliminated all bias in these proceedings?

8. Are you sure that you took the best possible course of action?

I rely on my personal experience and the following for addressing "problematic behaviors above:

Medical Staff Management Can Be Minefield
August 1, 2017
© 2021 Relias. All rights reserved.

Patient Satisfaction and Patient Complaints: The Long View, My 50 Years

Let us look at patient complaints. Based upon my fifty years of practice and researching the literature patient complaints can be based upon:

93. Personal Preference
94. Mistake
95. Mental Illness
96. Munchhausen Disorder
97. Secondary Gain
98. Criminal Behavior
99. Sport

Personal Preference:

Often the patient does not want the physician to be completing a progress note in the computer during the fact to face appointment.

Other patients want their statement entered into the record word for word as they speak to avoid distortion by memory.

I now make the following offer to the patient:

Do you want me to type your statements word for word while we take, or do you want me to take short notes and type a summary after the face-to-face meeting is completed?

The patient will choose between the following to statements for the record:

"I want my words typed into the note exactly as stated while we talk."

or:

"I want you to take short notes while we talk and write a brief summary after the face-to-face appointment is over."

Memories are reconstructed constructs and prone to error.

Patients often record doctor visits without the doctor's knowledge.

Federal law allows patients to tape record meetings without the doctor's knowledge. I always assume the patient is tape recording the meeting as it will not alter my treatment and I cannot search them for recording devices without their consent.

Surgeons have videotaped the patient giving consent to surgery including reviewing the risks and indicating that they understand the risk and accept the risks of the surgical procedure. They do this to avoid errors on the part of the patient and the physician based upon reconstructed memories.

I rely on:

The fallibility of memory in judicial processes: Lessons from the past and their modern consequences
Mark L. Howe, and Lauren M. Knott
Memory. 2015 Jul 4; 23(5): 633–656.
Published online 2015 Feb 23. doi: 10.1080/09658211.2015.1010709
PMCID: PMC4409058
PMID: 25706242

Complaints based upon mental illness.

The most famous case of complaints based upon mental illness is The McMartin preschool trial.

The McMartin preschool trial was based upon sexual abuse case in the 1980s.

The McMartin preschool trial was based upon a false complaint by a woman who suffered from paranoid schizophrenia.

False complaints based upon mental illness are common in mental health facilities.

I worked a State Hospital in Kalamazoo Michigan where false allegations were made almost daily, but each one was formally investigated by the State Police as required by law.

Complaints based upon secondary gain.

Patients will make complaints against the physician because:

1..They are addicted to drugs and alcohol and the physician refuses to prescribe addictive medications such as Xanax or Lunesta.

2.. The patient wants disability benefits, and the physician does not find a disability.

3.. The patient is subjective to criminal prosecution and the physician does not find the patient mentally incompetent to stand trial or insane to avoid conviction.

4..The patient wants addicting medications for resale and the physician refuses to prescribe addicting medications for chronic symptoms.

5..The patient wants time off from work and the physician does not find a basis to grant time off from work for medical reasons.

6.. Other reasons based upon divorce proceedings, child custody issues, lawsuits disputing wills, etc.

Complaints based upon criminal activities:

When I was working for the Michigan Department of Corrections from 1987 to 1991, they had a course entitled, "Anatomy of a Setup."

Anatomy of a Setup taught employees for the Michigan Department of Corrections how inmates would work as teams to trick a naive employee into making a series of rule violations. Then inmates would convince the employee that if they did not bring in drugs and engage in sex with the inmates the inmates would report the employee who would be prosecuted and go to prison.

This was not an idle threat as it is well known that prisoners have bribed employees into bringing drugs. The employees were then caught, prosecuted, and incarcerated.

In Michigan, the "Anatomy of a Setup," was taught by correctional officers who were trapped, but reported their issues to their superiors. They were not fired. They became credible trainers in the Anatomy of a Setup.

There are many reasons that a criminal will make false complaints or make threats of false complaints against physicians. Violence against health care workers is a crime, but rarely prosecuted.

I rely on:

Prevalence and policy of occupational violence against oral healthcare workers: systematic review and meta-analysis.
Binmadi, N.O., Alblowi, J.A.
BMC Oral Health 19, 279 (2019).
https://doi.org/10.1186/s12903-019-0974-3

Let us examine, "good faith," in making a record that supports a corrective action against a physician.

The U.S. Equal Employment Opportunity Commission, which was established by Title VII of the Civil Rights Act of 1964

The Civil Rights Act of 1964 prohibits discrimination and harassment of any type and affords equal employment opportunities to employees and applicants without regard to race, color, religion, sex, sexual orientation, gender identity or expression, pregnancy, age, national origin, disability status, genetic information, protected.

The United States Department of State has the following as a part of its policy:

"Any employee who believes he or she has been the target of sexual harassment is encouraged to inform the offending person orally or in writing that such conduct is unwelcome and offensive and must stop."

Why is this a policy?

The answer is that employees have encouraged a pattern of social conduct and then file a complaint. This is known as "entrapment."

The United State Department of Justice Defines Entrapment as:

645. ENTRAPMENT—ELEMENTS

Entrapment is a complete defense to a criminal charge, on the theory that "Government agents may not originate a criminal design, implant in an innocent person's mind the disposition to commit a criminal act, and then induce commission of the crime so that the Government may prosecute." Jacobson v. United States, 503 U.S. 540, 548 (1992). A valid entrapment defense has two related elements: (1) government inducement of the crime, and (2) the defendant's lack of predisposition to engage in the criminal conduct. Mathews v. United States, 485 U.S. 58, 63 (1988). Of the two elements, predisposition is by far the more important.

Inducement is the threshold issue in the entrapment defense. Mere solicitation to commit a crime is not inducement. Sorrells v. United States, 287 U.S. 435, 451 (1932). Nor does the government's use of artifice, stratagem, pretense, or deceit establish inducement. Id. at 441. Rather, inducement requires a showing of at least persuasion or mild coercion, United States v. Nations, 764 F.2d 1073, 1080 (5th Cir. 1985); pleas based on need, sympathy, or friendship, ibid.; or extraordinary promises of the sort "that would blind the ordinary person to his legal duties," United States v. Evans, 924 F.2d 714, 717 (7th Cir. 1991). See also United States v. Kelly, 748 F.2d 691, 698 (D.C. Cir. 1984) (inducement shown only if government's behavior was such that "a law-abiding citizen's will to obey the law could have been overborne"); United States v. Johnson, 872 F.2d 612, 620 (5th Cir. 1989) (inducement shown if government created "a substantial risk that an offense would be committed by a person other than one ready to commit it").

It is a tedious and uncertain task to prove or disprove "entrapment."

The obligation to object to "offensive behaviors," simplifies the process because behavior persisting after the notice is indicative of intent without inducement.

This obligation of notice with continuation of "problematic conduct" without corrective action is a factor in good faith.

If there is no notice with the opportunity of a good faith corrective action, it is difficult to support the assertion of good faith in applying any corrective action.

If there is no notice of "problematic behavior," with opportunity to make a corrective action there is insufficient basis to assert adequate training and supervision.

The issue of adequate training and supervision is an issue that allows the supervisor and the annual performance evaluation, the Executive Committee, the Credentialing Committee, the Chief of the Medical Staff, the Pharmaceutical Committee, the CEO and any other agent of the Medical Facility to be named as defendant for wrongful termination, libel, slander and a host of Complaints to be filed by the attorney with a fertile mind.

I have had patients that were the wives and children of police officers, ministers, psychiatrists, psychologists, and social workers.

Police officers, ministers, psychiatrists, psychologists, and social workers are preoccupied with good and evil and doing the right thing in difficult circumstances.

The children of these people often like to provoke their parents by breaking the law, sinning, violating social norms and even putting a tattoo of the bar code used in the jail during a period of incarceration on public display.

I had a lady bring her minister in for joint psychotherapy. What was peculiar was that the patient had no anxiety, anger, or depression. On the contrary the minister was very uncomfortable, and the patient was euphoric. I did not understand what was going on, but it just didn't seem right.

Later the minister was in the news for having sexual contact with a member of his ministry.

It all became clear. The practice of psychiatry is never simple or predictable.

This is merely an introduction to the many issues that intersect the concept of patient satisfaction.

This missive must end at some time, and I choose to end it here.

I am here to do no harm and help if I can.

Thank you for your time and attention.

William R. Yee M.D., J.D.
Board Certified Psychiatrist.
Practicing Medicine and Psychiatry without interruption since 1972 in Michigan, Indiana, Kentucky, California, and Texas
Recently licensed in Texas and excited about opportunities to live and practice in Texas, at your service.

"Pre-Existing text," includes names of symptoms, medical illnesses, medications, people, corporations, agencies, law cases, text of law cases, statutes, text of statutes, policies, the text of policies, the titles of articles, of books, the content of articles and books cited.

My copyright claim is a clam to the "original text," which is my personal experiences as described in the text above and my commentary on the names of symptoms, medical illnesses, medications, people, names of agencies, corporations, law cases, text of law cases, statutes, text of statutes, policies, the text of policies, the titles of articles, of books, the content of articles and books cited.